Dr Mike Dilke

CW00468256

STOP SNORING

...the easy way

And the real reasons you need to

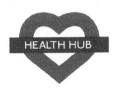

A Health Hub Publishing book
First published in Great Britain by Health Hub Books 2016
This edition published by Health Hub Books 2016-09-28
Copyright © Health Hub London

Cover and Design by SpiffingCovers Ltd.

To Veronica, Elizabeth, Julia, Holly, Ben, Max, Arthur, Charlotte, Olivia, Magnus and Roland

CONTENTS

Introduction

Much like drinking, smoking and junk food, snoring is a voluntary habit. You may not have consciously chosen to start but you can certainly make the choice to stop. Unlike the host of other voluntary habits and vices, research into the real effects of snoring on general wellbeing is virtually non-existent or not presented in a way that instigates discussion. Tales of friends and family shaking the rafters at night is a common narrative, and one that should prompt a deeper investigation into the associated health risks. Yet there seems to be little motivation to stop snoring other than social factors. The conversations that buck this trend are flooded with overly-complicated medical terminology, cause and effect jargon – completely inaccessible to the general community of sufferers.

The reality is that as a population we are blissfully unaware of the real dangers of snoring and the consuming effects it has on every aspect of one's life. This book presents a study into snoring, a targeted summary of the threats to one's wellbeing and a simple daily exercise routine to stop snoring all together.

We follow a model which argues a person is only motivated to stop a voluntary habit if they:

- Have a useable understanding of their condition
- Understand how this effects "them" and "their life"
- Have easy to follow action points which yield great results quickly

In chapters 1-3 we discuss the anatomical evolutions that set the stage for the snoring epidemic and investigate the differing levels of its clinical severity. We also introduce a key theme of the book: that snoring prevents our natural phases of sleep and the essential sleep cycles.

Chapters 4-7 answer the question "how does this affect me?" based on an understanding of "which factors are most important to me?" We analyse the real effects of snoring on your professional success, relationships, sex life, health, fitness and finally on your vanity goals.

In Chapter 8 we outline an easy to implement 5-minute routine to life-hack yourself back into deep, restful sleep at night, and into a healthy, energetic and happy life every day.

Chapter 1

The Real Dangers of Snoring

The answer to the question "what is the problem with snoring?" will almost always relate, at least partially, to social stigma. In every group or family there is at least one member who is infamous for being a snorer. That person is usually male, and typically fathers, husbands and boyfriends whose nightly routines are the topic of lifelong ridicule. Many men find this reputation embarrassing and can become defensive about the subject, finding it uncomfortable to discuss in public what is considered to be a particularly unattractive habit.

A common assumption is that snoring is the pastime of men, and whilst they account for the majority of snorers worldwide, a whopping 20% of adult women are also severe snorers. The stigma attached is in general far worse for women. Snoring can therefore be an incredibly sensitive topic and in many social situations is out of bounds when it comes to poking fun.

It is easy to understand why the problem of snoring is regarded as unattractive and disruptive when one considers the loudness of a snore that the average adult produces.

The level of noise generated by snoring lies on the range of 60 to 100 decibels[1]. Even at the lower end of the scale, the average volume can be compared to the loudness of a household vacuum cleaner. The more extreme cases approach the volume you would expect from a chainsaw or even a motorbike.

Little wonder then that humiliation and shame are the most common theme in answering "what is wrong with snoring?" Equally a number of books on snoring cite this as the sole reason for taking action, with numerous references to snoring causing the breakdown of marriages and preventing relationships from starting altogether. Again this is understandable but it ignores a greater concern. Part of the purpose of this book is to shed light on the much under- publicised and far more alarming danger that 60% of the population face as they drift off to sleep.

Even mild snoring presents the real dangers of a prolonged nocturnal breathing disorder which has significant effects on many aspects of the healthy body and mind. This is well understood by the medical community, but advice and treatment tend to focus on purely medical aspects. Whilst surgery and ventilation aids have a real place in the treatment of snoring, they are an extreme step, especially when simple but effective measures have often not been tried.

1: *There have been a number of cases in which decibel readings have topped 115 decibels, about the same volume as a jet fighter plane.*

This book aims to simplify the treatment of a common and often debilitating medical problem. We follow a simple model:

- Create awareness
- Embed "how this applies to me"
- Give the steps needed to act and help resolve the problem

Chapter 2

What is Snoring?

Snoring, by its medical definition, is called "stertor". This means noisy breathing. It happens whilst we are asleep because that's when the airway collapses and becomes partially blocked. The noise of snoring is produced from a reduction in muscle tone causing structures in the throat to start to flap - rather like a sail or flag flapping when the wind reaches a certain speed. It's all to do with turbulent air flow and resonance. There are three parts of our throat which tend to flap because they are not firmly fixed to anything. They are the soft palate, the uvula and the epiglottis. As these structures flap about under the correct conditions of high flow, turbulent breathing, they trap air against the back wall of the throat for a split second, causing a very high pressure build up and subsequent sound wave, just like clapping your hands together. You might ask why this doesn't happen when you have high flow breathing from exercise - that's because muscle tone holds everything in place, including the soft palate, uvula and epiglottis.

Normal breathing while we are awake also doesn't tend to cause snoring, as it is relatively low energy, and our breathing tube is held open widely by the muscles of the throat. That's what we mean by muscle tone. When we tense our arm or stomach muscles and they become hard and firm, that's an example of high muscle tone. It is obviously much harder to make a hard muscle flap than a soft, low tone one.

When the airway collapses due to low muscle tone, oxygen levels drop a little, which is registered in the brain. This causes a signal to go to the lungs so that more effort is put into breathing and enough air is shifted to restore normal oxygenation. The lungs duly comply, increasing their force, causing an increase in the speed of flow so that enough air is moved in and out. Think of a small but fast flowing river, with the same net flow as a wide and slow-moving one.

Why Do We Snore?

In the living world, only Homo sapiens (humans) snore as a result of their natural development. Some animals make loud breathing sounds, particularly when asleep, but this is because of characteristics bred into them, like the British bulldog or an overweight family dog. Snoring is not a good characteristic in terms of survival in the wild as it can alert a predator to the presence of an easy, sleeping target.

Humans snore mainly because of speech and posture. The evolution of speech meant that a number of changes had to happen to the throat, so that the rudimentary grunts and noises of our chimpanzee ancestors could become the wide range complex framework of interaction we call speech.

Firstly, the breathing tube had to become longer because the larynx (voice box), where coarse sound is produced, had to be separated from the mouth, where sound is made into speech. This separation is called the throat, or in medical terms, the oropharynx. As a result the throat is a muscular tube that can collapse at night as it is not held open by bone or cartilage, unlike the mouth or larynx.

Secondly, for range of speech the tongue needed to change its relationship within the mouth, sitting further back. This caused narrowing of the gap between the tongue and the back of the throat[2] which when combined with a marginal collapse of the throat, triggers turbulent airflow and snoring.

Much like speech, the evolution of posture caused changes that trigger snoring. The most notable change was walking on two feet. The upright nature of this meant that the relationship of the skull and the throat altered, with the throat being located more centrally under the skull, rather than being further forward. This narrowed any available throat space, as it was confined against the hard tissue of the spine. Narrowing of this

2: In medical speech this is called "the retrolingual space."

area again made blockage easier to occur, especially at night when muscle tone was lost in sleep.

We have a built-in predilection to snore due to our development of speech and upright posture. Yet not all of us snore. Why are some people different to others? Firstly, it may simply be due to the shape of one's face, skull and neck. There are certain features that people are born with, which make them more susceptible to snoring. These include a significant lower jaw underbite, a small mouth, a large tongue, a small lower jaw or a misshapen epiglottis. Then there are other acquired reasons for snoring, like a blocked nose, large tonsils, long soft palate and cysts or lumps in the throat. Finally, obesity is another cause of snoring simply because the weight of fat in the neck can collapse the airway.

Nevertheless, in all these cases we only make snoring sounds at night when asleep, no matter how bad our anatomy is. So, what happens in sleep to trigger snoring?

Sleep

Sleep occurs so that the body can refresh itself, both physically and mentally. There are two main types of sleep, REM and non-REM. The abbreviation REM stands for rapid eye movement, and if you look into someone's eyes by lifting up the eyelids while they are in this phase of sleep, the eyes will be flickering all over the place. Different phases of sleep are associated with loss of muscle tone which causes snoring.

There are 4 stages of non-REM sleep and one true REM sleep.

Non-REM sleep phases:
- Drifting off to sleep and can easily be woken
- Mental slowdown in preparation for deep, non-REM sleep
- Transitional phase, moving into deep sleep, when muscle tone is lost and the body starts regenerating
- True deep sleep when most of the regeneration process occurs, and when muscle tone remains very low

It is essential that the body achieves stage 4 non-REM sleep, as this is when we begin to dream, and it is only at this point the body begins the process of restful rejuvenation and repair.

REM Sleep

True REM sleep is when we do most of our dreaming and is associated with a marked loss in muscle tone. REM sleep stimulates the brain regions used in learning and is essential for normal brain development during infancy, which is why children have a higher proportion of REM sleep than adults[3]. Lack of REM sleep can be disastrous and throughout this book we discuss how this can lead to irreversible damage to the body, serious psychiatric issues and ultimately death. The general recommendation is that we achieve seven to eight hours of sleep per night. Interestingly, only two hours or so of this is stage 4 non-REM and REM sleep – the bit you actually need. Those who can survive on a few hours' sleep at night are likely to be able to skip stages 1-3 and go straight to stage 4 non-REM sleep and REM sleep.

Sleep Apnoea

Finally, many of you reading this article will have heard of, probably literally, snoring. Most of you won't know what sleep apnoea is. Apnoea means "no breathing", so sleep apnoea is when you stop breathing at night, while you are asleep.

Snoring, when left untreated, may progress to sleep apnoea over the passage of time. Approximately 40% of males over the age of 35 snore regularly, of these 2% have sleep apnoea. At the age of 65, 70% of males snore regularly and 10% have sleep apnoea.

When you have fully-developed sleep apnoea, your blood oxygen concentration can regularly drop below

3: *Brain Basics: Understanding Sleep, National Institute of Neurological Disorder and Stroke, 2014*

90% and it usually runs at around 98-99%. This low oxygen supply can go on for a large proportion of a patient's sleep time.

This means your organs are deprived of oxygen for significant periods of time at night, and if their oxygen supply is already a bit precarious, as in patients with furring of the arteries (atherosclerosis), then this loss of oxygen can become critical. Sleep apnoea is associated with all sorts of other medical problems, from heart attacks in the middle of the night, to impotence, lack of concentration, poor memory, diabetes and blood pressure. People with sleep apnoea usually have a score above 10 on the Epworth Sleepiness Scale[4]. Sleep apnoea is best diagnosed by overnight pulse oximetry using a simple finger probe.

Traditional Treatment

The treatment of snoring is to unblock the airway. Methods include Continuous Positive Airway Pressure (CPAP) which involves having a ventilator fitted over the face at night, which forces air into the lungs, causing the airway to be stretched open.

Treatment can also mean having a tooth splint fitted to the upper and lower jaw at night, holding the lower jaw

4: The Epworth Sleepiness Scale (ESS) is a scale intended to measure daytime sleepiness by use of a very short questionnaire. This can be helpful in diagnosing sleep disorders. It was introduced in 1991 by Dr Murray Johns of Epworth Hospital in Melbourne, Australia.

in a forward position, which in turn pulls the tongue forward and opens the airway at the back of the tongue, the most common site for airway obstruction at night. Otherwise, surgery can be performed to improve the airway, to reduce the tonsils (laser tonsillectomy), shrink the soft palate (laser palatoplasty) or open up the nose (septoplasty).

Weight loss is also a common recommendation. Your body mass index (BMI) should be less than 30. To calculate your BMI take your weight in kilogrammes, and divide it by your height in metres, squared (i.e. your height in metres multiplied by your height in metres). Losing weight both reduces the oxygen requirement of the body, meaning you breathe more lightly, and reduces the bulk of the neck, which means there is less pressure on the airway so it obstructs less easily.

As with most diseases, self-help can often play a major role, bearing in mind:

- Untreated sleep apnoea can seriously damage your health.
- Untreated snoring can seriously damage your wealth.
- This book has been produced as there is no thorough, concise regime to treat snoring at home by non-medical means currently available.
- Now we are going to tell you how this applies to you, and what you personally can do about it.

Chapter 3

Tiredness, Exhaustion and Burnout

The city never sleeps and neither, it seems, does its workers. Long hours are now a staple of the glamourous city life, with many films and TV shows depicting its protagonists in late night office scenarios, sporting crystal glasses of whiskey and wearing £5000 suits. For those that live this lifestyle however the truth is that 90 hour weeks only promise prestige and riches in the future, if you forego your personal life now, mortgaging your future. Abstaining from social life is one thing but the exhaustion of such unforgiving hours at the office is far more concerning and would have most asking "is this really worth it?"

Aiming for three to four hours sleep a night has become the norm for many, especially in the banking and technology sectors where there are enough sub-30-year-old millionaires to keep a steady flow of interest from the young talent following suit. But what if you aren't actually getting three to four hours of restorative, Stage 4 non-REM and REM sleep? We are told that on average the partner of a snorer loses 90 minutes of sleep per night. So that equates to a maximum of two and half hours restorative sleep if you happen to share your bed with a snorer.

If you are the one snoring and working on this time schedule, even two and a half hours of restorative sleep a night is optimistic and therefore incredibly dangerous. The sufferer is building a continuous backlog of sleep debt which becomes impossible to repay, blindly passing through days on end without getting sufficient rest. The health risks involved will be highlighted shortly but it is amazing that businesses that operate like this don't address this problem. The raw facts are that their people will get less done, less effectively and need more time to do it if they are exhausted. This quickly becomes what is now widely recognised as "burnout".

What do top companies want from their people? Why would they want to create a population that without proper sleep are guaranteed to have slower reaction times, reduced accuracy, cognitive impairment, become irritable easily and experience serious lapses in memory, even suffering permanent memory loss? This method is clearly unsustainable for all involved as the employee struggles and the employer is destined to lose good people.

Remember that the epidemic, and it is becoming just that, of burnout in the professional considers only those who are aiming to get two to three hours of restorative sleep per night. If you are a snorer the available time to fall into deep mental sleep repair is significantly decreased.

Using the survival mantra of the three 3s, one cannot survive for longer than:

- 3 minutes without air
- 3 days without water
- 3 weeks without food

With respect to sleep, there have been numerous cases and indeed challenges to measure the extremes in time a subject is able to stay awake, some reaching the outer limits of a full week. Whilst the subjects did not die in these cases, science tells us that after 72 hours the body will start to display irreparable side effects[5], and a complete absence of sleep will ultimately kill you. The authors argue that the three 3s of survival need updating and re-launching as the four 3s to include: 3 days without sleep[6]

On Thursday 15 August 2013 the body of Mortiz Erhardt, a 21-year-old intern for Merrill Lynch, was found in the shower at home after a 72-hour straight stint at his City of London placement. In order to impress his employer, as is expected for competitive jobs in finance, he had worked day and night for three days, following what has become known as "The Magic Roundabout" regime. Graduates on this regime hail

5: http://sleepjunkies.com/features/sleep-deprivation-and-torture-a-brief-history/
6: Of course all the 3s are in some form subjective with many instances of extreme cases, for example, people holding their breath for 10 minutes or indeed forgoing sleep for a week. The point is that whilst a bullet to the head might not kill you, let's work with the assumption that it will.

taxis back to their apartments from the office around 5am each morning. The taxi driver waits outside whilst the intern washes and changes clothes and then drives them immediately back to the office at dawn. An inquest revealed that Erhardt died from a seizure thought to be induced by exhaustion[7].

Aside from the miserable existence, it is amazing to think that these types of periods of uninterrupted sleep fit those classed as "Sleep Deprivation Torture" by the CIA[8].

In the "Whitehall II Study", British researchers looked at how sleep patterns affected the mortality of more than 10,000 British civil servants over two decades. The results, published in 2007, showed that those who had cut their sleep from seven to five hours or less a night nearly doubled their risk of death from all causes. In particular, lack of sleep doubled the risk of death from cardiovascular disease.

Clearly, extreme lack of sleep is highly dangerous and undesirable, however the effects of seemingly little loss of sleep must also not be underestimated. Sufficient stage 4 non-REM and REM sleep is key to longevity.

7: https://www.theguardian.com/business/2013/nov/22/moritz-erhadt-death-exhaustion-parents-bank-america-epilepsy
8: https://www.theguardian.com/us-news/2014/dec/09/cia-torture-methods-waterboarding-sleep-deprivation

Chapter 4

Obesity and the Associated Risks

It is not the intention of this book to associate snoring with obesity exclusively. However obesity, defined by a BMI greater than 30, can be part of the problem.

So, what do we know of obesity alone? Being overweight is no different to any other bad habit. Whilst you might be genetically predisposed to retaining weight (the big boned argument), the choice to consume high calorie, nutritionally devoid foods is entirely yours to make.

The three most recognised risks of obesity are coronary heart disease, high blood pressure and stroke.

Obesity is related to these conditions because it is associated with the build-up of deposits or "plaque" within blood vessels.

This causes narrowing of the blood vessels and a reduction in the supply of oxygen, which limits the amount of blood that can be pumped by the heart around your body. This is what we mean by heart disease. Left untreated, further build-up within the arteries will likely lead to heart failure or heart attack.

It follows that any build-up creates a point of resistance for the natural flow of blood through the body. The increase in peripheral resistance leads to high blood pressure. Your body is therefore in constant overdrive and this is a key factor in the rise of all other obesity-related risks[9].

The logical next step here is the body having to give in to the pressure you are putting it under. Prolonged internal stress and strain within an artery can cause breaks and ruptures which trigger a clotting cascade which in turn leads to the formation of a clot. This can block the flow much like standing on a garden hose, restricting the stream of oxygenated blood almost entirely. Very simply, if that rupture occurs in close proximity to your brain, the lack of oxygen available will cause a stroke, if it is in the heart, then it will cause a heart attack.

And Now Add Snoring...

Information about the dangerous habits that will hasten the onset of the above ailments is becoming more and more available. In particular the risks associated with being overweight and also being a smoker, drinker and living a generally sedentary life. It is hugely important to add snoring to this list of dangerous, voluntary habits.

9: Type 2 diabetes, abnormal blood fats, metabolic syndrome, cancer, osteoarthritis, sleep apnoea, obesity hypoventilation syndrome, reproductive problems, gallstones and death.

Although we have discussed the dangers of obstructive sleep apnoea, importantly it is the common snorer, one in ten women and one in four men, who is also at risk. Sleep apnoea causes constant and regular breaks in the necessary in and outflow of oxygen through the airways. These regular stoppages require the heart to work harder as there is less available oxygenated blood flowing through the body. Working harder means a rise in blood pressure, in other words heavy snorers and sleep apnoeics are once again at risk of hypertension.

It is important to realise the dual effect of being overweight and an acute snorer, beyond the relation of one causing the other. Given the statistics, adult men and women are very likely to already be snorers before their BMI reaches the point of plaque build-up. Therefore high blood pressure is already incipient within the body, making the dangers of obesity far more real, and the likelihood of them occurring all the more quickly.

In summary it should be widely acknowledged that heavy snoring, or apnoea, coupled with obesity sets the way for a perfect storm.

The exercises in Chapter 8 will not entirely resolve snoring that is partially caused by a person's weight. However an increase in muscle tone in the three areas of the throat and mouth outlined will be of significant benefit. The exercises should become routine immediately, in combination with those that support losing weight. Over time weight loss and increased muscle tone in the throat and mouth will meet in the middle, and life changing health benefits will follow.

The central theme of this book is to introduce the fact that everything in your life is negatively affected by snoring and this is why you must take action to stop.

Chapter 5

Relationships and Sex

Perhaps the most widely documented side effect of snoring is the bearing it has on others, in particular your partner. This marks the point one's night time routine goes beyond social stigma and becomes an occurrence of the everyday.

The most extreme cases are those we hear about, exemplified by an Australian study in which 30 of 500 women cited snoring as the sole cause for the breakdown and end of their marriages. When 6% of marriages break down because of a largely voluntary habit, one would think the motivation to act would be close behind. However the trend is nowhere to be seen. If the threat of losing your partner is not reason enough to change, then let's work backwards and analyse the effects of snoring on different elements of a relationship.

Sleeping Separately

As discussed, consistently disrupted sleep affects our ability to operate rationally during waking hours. It's not hard to imagine the trajectory couples follow when both parties are tired and irritated due to a lack of restful sleep. The most common solution to this is sleeping in separate bedrooms. At face value it is encouraging that a couple would take this measure to maintain a happy relationship. However, many studies into sleep psychology paint a different picture, as impairments through lack of sleep in the snorer will ultimately lead to major resentments and even depression. In recent history relationships and certainly marriage are defined by the sharing of a bed. In the same Australian study mentioned above 40% of women interviewed now slept in separate bedrooms to their partners.

Luxury bed companies in the United States have seen this as a real opportunity, and we entered the dawn of the "snoring room" or "second master suite". The argument is that with increased wealth comes a need for a greater level of comfort. Therefore it is essential that successful and "would-be" successful men and women of the future sleep uninterrupted. Whilst the sentiment of this argument is undeniable, the reality is that snoring is a habit which means that natural measures to stem and even stop snoring should be adopted long before sleeping apart is ever considered.

Sex

If the threat of divorce and sleeping separately are still not enough to motivate you into stopping snoring then one much under-discussed side effect almost certainly will, namely:

Snoring and its effect on your sex life
The most common reason male fitness enthusiasts give for not using steroids is invariably not those you would have assumed: enlargement of vital organs, heart failure, fear of needles, drug induced rage or even death. It is actually the rumours and stories of a reduction in the size of the testicles that prevent most from taking steroids.

Imagine then if it were widely accepted that snoring affected your manhood in exactly the same way. A huge industry would appear to stop and prevent us from snoring almost overnight. In reality this is not so far from the truth. You might find it shocking that snoring can and does cause a range of sexual dysfunctions.

The first dysfunction is related to the bedroom environment of tired couples and the types of resentment we have outlined, which prevents them from sleeping together. Not only that, even before the point of not sleeping together 21% of women whose partners were also mild snorers said that this caused a major loss of intimacy in their relationship.

Men and women who are deprived of sleep report lower libidos and less interest in sex due to depleted energy, sleepiness and increased tension. In a study of men suffering from severe sleep apnoea, nearly half of the men secreted abnormally low levels of testosterone, the main male sex hormone, during the night[10].

We find that one fact, however, is far more effective at calling couples to action. Men especially are alarmed to learn that snoring can have a direct effect on their ability to maintain an erection. The science is simple. As we have discussed snoring and apnoea cause high blood pressure. High pressure in the arteries causes internal damage, making them thicker. This restricts blood flow around the body, including to the penis, causing erectile dysfunction or impotence.

Snoring alone can prevent men from achieving and maintaining an erection long enough for sexual function. However, coupled with a host of other mitigating effects we once again find ourselves at the eye of a perfect storm. We have outlined how interrupted sleep through snoring can cause increased stress and anxiety, both of which are concurrent themes in diagnosing erectile dysfunction. These psychological effects on sexual performance will often be the hardest to shake.

Most men assume that there is something beyond their control which increases anxiety prior to going into the bedroom. The constant concern of "underperformance"

10: Omar Burschtin and Jing Wang, 'Testosterone Deficiency and Sleep Apnea', Urologic Clinics of North America, May 2016, Volume 43, Issue 2, pp. 233–237 can leave men with an inability to maintain an erection for months, even years, driven solely by their mindset. Of course the effects of erectile dysfunction doesn't only affect the men in a relationship. The psychological trauma of being seemingly unattractive to your partner by being a snorer has often irrevocable consequences for women as well. This apparent lack of sexual interest has been identified as having major effects on self-confidence and happiness. A woman's natural response is to internalise this problem and assuming "it's all my fault" can also cause the onset of depression.

If only couples knew that the dysfunctions they suffer from are in large part due to the chosen, voluntary habits they have in day to day life.

Once again the exercises that follow may break one's current routine, albeit marginally, in terms of actually having to do them and embedding them as part of the everyday. However they are infinitesimal when we consider the extremes that couples, partners and individuals are putting themselves through on a daily basis because of their snoring.

Chapter 6

Health, Fitness and Vanity Goals

We have entered an age where a person's key motivations in life are determined by the effect they have on our health, fitness and appearance. The latest anti-oxidant juice, cleanse or workout routines emerge on almost a daily basis and those in pursuit of physical and aesthetic perfection rush to adopt them as part of their everyday life.

Bad habits are something that these groups of people find easy to cut out. Whether it be alcohol, smoking, fatty foods or dairy. Abstaining from the temptation is worth the results they will see physically. However, it is interesting to see that snoring is never highlighted as one such undesirable, voluntary habit.

You would imagine that the key reason health conscious teenagers give for not smoking and drinking is because of the multitude of health risks associated with them. Interestingly however, they are far more concerned with premature ageing of the skin and teeth discolouration than they are with lung cancer and liver disease. Whilst this is a strange way to come round to abstinence, any thought process that makes it easy to stop these voluntary habits is a good thing.

Sleep or rather "beauty sleep" is a concurrent theme in most health and beauty regimes. This is particularly encouraging as nearly all workouts and nutritional advice recommend proper restful sleep as key to maximising your results. The rule of thumb for nutrition is that getting in proper shape involves 20% of your time in the gym and 80% of your time in the kitchen. This is a great mantra as it points to the natural ability of the body to restore and improve itself when operating at its natural peak through the nutrients you put into it.

A much under-discussed element is just how important the restful sleep part of this routine is. Moreover it's about how you make sure you are maximising restful sleep and understanding those things which prevent you from getting it. Based on our research we would like to see a shift in understanding so that the optimum breakdown of importance is perceived as:

- 20% in the gym
- 40% in the kitchen
- 40% in deep restful sleep

Getting to this point will take increased awareness of sleep but more importantly about the effects of disruptive sleep caused by snoring. What follows is a brief run through of the physical limitations and effects snoring has on your appearance.

Snoring Makes You Gain weight!

Lack of sleep stimulates appetite. The most popular workouts cite the difference between those people who secure six hours of sleep a night versus those that manage eight to nine hours. A key difference between these groups is the increase in cravings for high carbohydrate and high-fat foods in the sleep-deprived group, as they try to ward off the feelings of sleepiness by getting a sugar hit to keep active when actually they just want to sleep, not eat. This is like the much-needed coffee or doughnut that many indulge in during the later stages of the afternoon whilst at work. Your fatigue is signalling the body to act with what it thinks is the best course to keep you alert.

The important thing to bear in mind here is the likelihood that most acute snorers are unable to achieve even close to the lower target of six hours of restful sleep per night. The cravings therefore become harder to fight the less rest you get. The fact that you are a snorer means you are faced with bad eating choices for much more of the time as your body is under increased fatigue more often.

Snoring Ages the Skin!

A constant battle in the world of cosmetics is the need to fight and reverse the signs of ageing. The aim is also to mask or reduce fine lines, sallow skin and dark circles around the eye. As mentioned above it is common knowledge that a host of other voluntary habits cause these tell-tale signs of ageing and as a result we have seen a steady reduction in a number of smokers and regular drinkers. The reality is that creams, potions and pills are not the only (very expensive) solution to this. Early deleterious effects on our appearance are in most cases the result of our voluntary habits. Stop the habit and the body's natural defences will kick into action and dark circles for example, will be a thing of the past. The problem with the voluntary habit of snoring is that it is incredibly effective at not allowing our natural defences to work optimally – as the sleep debt increases so does our inability to pay it back. This is because in the restorative stages of sleep (stage 4 non-REM and REM sleep) the body releases growth hormones which are key to the rebuilding of damaged and aged cells in the body, and especially the face. Lack of sleep made worse by snoring means that far too little of these vital hormones are released and the skin is never entirely rejuvenated.

Interestingly it follows that those who suffer from skin conditions and whose skins' defences are already low, take far longer to heal, if at all, due to lack of proper sleep. In contrast those that get sufficient REM sleep recover much quicker from skin ailments and the effects of sun damage and irritation.

The body will naturally repair itself, so before synthetic creams and expensive methods are adopted we must first address those factors which keep our bodies from working as they should. Paying more attention to sleep, and snoring in particular, can only help successful rejuvenation to take effect.

Chapter 7

Sleep Hygiene

Not everyone who snores is mortgaging their future like the city executives mentioned earlier. Most snorers have the option of maximising good sleep but fail to do so.

These people are not taking the correct basic steps to reduce or even stop their condition by understanding proper sleep hygiene. The term hygiene brings to mind a focus on personal cleanliness prior to bed, maybe fresh bedding or an ordered, clutter-free bedroom. Whilst these elements would help ensure a better night's rest in a practical sense, it's actually what they contribute to that defines what is meant by proper sleep hygiene: a routine which prepares us mentally for healthy sleep and daytime alertness[11].

The steps outlined above certainly contribute to making a cleaner, calmer environment which helps clear the mind. However, it's what we do with this mental preparedness that is most important. One key observation is the likelihood that rather than seeing our bed as a place for rest, we commonly see it as an extension of the living space. Watching TV and movies,

11: https://sleepfoundation.org

playing games, reading and eating are now very normal activities that take place in the bedroom and this needs to change.

This routine is just as relevant to non-snorers as snorers, but the point here is when the latter is already up against a huge reduction in the available restorative hours, following proper sleep hygiene is going to help.

However, taking on too many changes in any new regime is destined for failure, so if you are only going to do one thing, keep your pre-bed routine the same and just follow the exercises in Chapter 8. If you have really committed to the idea of getting more rest and increasing daily alertness the list below serves as a starting point. Pick one and stick to it, thereby making it a habit. Then incorporate the second and so on and so forth. You will very quickly see a big change – guaranteed.

Blueprint for Good Sleep Hygiene

Don't eat high-calorie meals close to bedtime and be aware of what is in your snacks and evening treats, for example chocolate contains caffeine.

Cut out stimulants such as tea and coffee[12] two to three hours prior to bed.

Try and avoid strenuous exercise in the evening, and take it instead in the morning or afternoon[13].

Get outside in the day! Maximising your exposure to natural light will help regulate your internal body clock and help with the forming of a day and night regime.

Don't nap in the day, even if you're tired. Get the regime right and you will see a rise in your energy levels so midday napping becomes a thing of the past.

Turn off all laptops, TVs, radios and close this book at least one hour before sleep. Mental stimulation will prevent you from entering restorative sleep.

This list is by no means exhaustive but highlights some key first steps in getting sleep hygiene right. The idea here is to redefine the bedroom as a place we associate predominantly with sleep.

12: A common misconception exists around caffeine levels in flavoured or therapeutic tea blends. Jasmine and green tea, for example, have higher caffeine levels than coffee. Also be aware that the terms "decaffeinated" and "alcohol free" are used for marketing purposes. The former actually means reduced caffeine, not no caffeine. The latter typically contains 0.5% alcohol.
13: Yoga and other light stretching regimes are fine for the evening and can actually assist the preparation for restful sleep.

Chapter 8
The Workouts

Notice

If you have jumped straight to this section of the book then welcome! The mentality for a quick and easy fix is something that we anticipated which is why the workouts are not only short, but also why this chapter is usable without reading any other element of this guide. However, achieving the maximum results and committing to real everyday action can only come with sufficient awareness of "why it is important for me to stop snoring". Therefore please take an additional 10 minutes to flick back to the chapter or chapters that relate most to you.

The "Only Way to Stop Snoring Permanently Workout" draws on a wealth of existing tongue, soft palate and jaw muscle routines, but consolidates their best parts into one 5 minute workout we have designed specifically to treat snoring.

As with any strength training the more you do with correct form, the better your results. It is clear, however, that it is unrealistic to expect snorers to adopt a new 60-minute training regime[14] and perform

14: www.torbayandsouthdevon.nhs.uk/uploads/23558.pdf

it every night. We have learned the lessons of the dental hygiene industry who ask patients to simply brush their teeth twice a day for two minutes. The benefits of proper oral hygiene are easy to find and yet one in four adults don't brush twice a day, with one in ten not brushing at all15. If adults are unable to adopt a routine as simple as a four-minute brushing habit, then the likelihood of them incorporating a 30-60 minute additional programme for snoring won't ever get off the ground.

The workout is designed as if you are going to do the bare minimum. If there has to be just one workout to help you stop snoring permanently – make it this one. Hopefully by this point you know what snoring is and the effect it has on your life so let's solve it.

This workout focuses on three key areas:
- The tongue
- The soft palate
- The lower throat

As we have discussed above these are the central points that relax during sleep, closing and restricting the natural in-and-out flow of air through the mouth and nose, causing us to snore. Exercising the muscles in these areas reduces the restriction of air flow and will ultimately allow the newly firm muscles to hold

15: http://www.nationalsmilemonth.org/facts-figures/

themselves naturally in place, without relaxing. Successfully targeting these muscle groups is safe, inexpensive and effective[16], and in this format can be easily incorporated into your everyday life.

Strength Training

The methods of increasing strength and tone are simple and effective. It is essentially yoga for the mouth as it involves stretching and positional training. With all of these exercises the emphasis is on fast repetition, rather than slow high effort as this will cause bulk rather than tone which is undesirable when trying to keep the airways open.

In particular we are aiming to target the base of the tongue and muscles that constitute the upper airway. These soft tissues are relaxed and floppy when asleep due to reduced muscle tone, so it is essential to tighten them and reduce the amount of relaxation. Tightening will also decrease the amount of vibration since the soft tissue is unable to flap as readily during sleep. The first results you will see, or rather hear, when getting this workout right is a reduction in the volume of snoring. A detailed analysis into tongue and mouth exercises showed that patients can reduce their snoring volume

16: http://www.huffingtonpost.com/2015/06/25/how-to-stop-snoring-_n_7657348.html

by nearly 60%[17], and reduce the frequency of snoring by 39%[18].

Treatments of this kind are in their infancy but are revolutionising the way specialists treat their patients. Out with gadgets, sprays and clips and in with exercise. "This…demonstrates a promising, non-invasive treatment for large populations suffering from snoring, the snorers and their bed partners, that are largely omitted from research and treatment…Frankly, this will change the advice that I give to my patients who snore. And that's a lot of people."

Barbara Phillips, MD, FCCP, President-Designate, American College of Chest Physicians and Medical Director, Sleep Laboratory at the University of Kentucky College of Medicine.

Tightening the Tongue

The tongue is the key area for upper airway obstruction in snorers. More specifically, the area in and around the back of the tongue, also referred to as the retrolingual space. Any tone and strength increase at this point helps to bring the tongue forward and widen this space, reducing frequency and volume in snoring.

17: V. Leto, F. Kayamor, M.I. Montes, 'Effects of Oropharyngeal Exercises on Snoring: A Randomised Trial', Chest, 2015, Volume 148, Issue 3, pp. 14-2953
18: http://www.medicaldaily.com/cures-snoring-mouth-and-tongue-exercises-thatll-help-you-stop-snoring-better-sleep-332444

Tongue Extenders

Stick your tongue out straight as far as it will go. Touch the tip of your tongue to the end of your nose, then depress it to touch your chin, then move it to touch your left then right cheek.

Repeat quickly 10 times.

Tongue Curls

Move the tip of your tongue backwards in your mouth, so it curls over towards the soft palate. Stretch it as far back as it will go, then bring it forward to touch the back of the upper teeth.

Repeat quickly 15 times.

Hummers

Grip the tip of your tongue gently between your teeth. Make a humming sound, starting deep then increase in frequency until it is as high pitched as you can make it.

Repeat 10 times.

Tightening the Soft Palate

The soft palate is one of the main parts of the throat involved in snoring. It is a soft, mobile structure, sitting in the back of the mouth and can flap about which is what snoring noise is caused by. Its main function is to prevent food and drink entering the nose when eating or drinking.

This is a key area as shown by the many operations devised to shorten and stiffen the soft palate in snorers. Far better to use regular muscular training as described, rather than embark on a series of painful and expensive surgeries.

Mouth Stretchers (The Hippo)
Open your mouth as widely as you can and say, "Ahhhhhhhhh," for 20 seconds. Use a timer.
Repeat once.

Intervals
With your mouth closed, try and breathe in sharply through the nose. The sensation you will feel is a raising of the roof of the mouth. You may snort a bit.
Do this rapidly in 4 sets of 5 repetitions each, with a 5-second break between each set.

Extended half intervals
With your tongue protruding out of your mouth as far as it will go, take long deep breaths in and out of your nose.
Repeat 20 times.

Tightening the Lower Throat
The throat, or oropharynx, is a muscular tube running from the back of the mouth to the voice box. It is easily collapsed by factors such as external pressure (fat neck) and increased respiratory effort (breathing in). Increasing tone and strength here helps hold the airway open during sleep.

Gulpers
Swallow 10 times consecutively with your mouth closed. Make it as forceful as you can (this is a lot harder than you might think, please take your time and persevere).

Pitchers
With your tongue poking out as far as it will go, take a deep breath in and make a high pitched noise, like air gargling. Do this for 30 seconds. It can be at low volume so you don't wake the rest of the house!

Boas
Complete a standard swallow motion, but make it last 5 seconds. Hold as much pressure as possible in the throat throughout and repeat 5 times. The key to getting this exercise right is a slow, controlled swallow.

With practice you will become quicker and better at doing these exercises.

The All in One Shortcut

As commitment is essential to getting the results that you want, those people who struggle with the full routine at least need somewhere to start. We have therefore devised a short, effective but fun introductory exercise to get people going. Although using this exercise alone will have a number of snoring benefits, for maximum results we must recommend that you ultimately adopt the nine daily exercises outlined above.

Cop-Out Easy Adopter:

Start with your mouth open as wide as it can go and tongue protruding out forwards as far as it will go. Whilst holding these two positions begin moving the extended tongue in an up, down, side to side movement. After two revolutions of these movements begin humming your national anthem in as deep a pitch as you can and continue until the end of the song or for at least two minutes, whichever comes first!

Chapter 9

Pledge and Intentions

By this point you should: understand what snoring is, how the dangers apply to you and your life, and finally you should be primed to make these simple exercises part of your every day to stop snoring. However good intentions have a bad reputation as, for example, people who form New Year's resolutions earn at best a sympathetic smile when they announce their heroic intentions[19].

Most people that set goals fail. Not by trying and missing the mark (this would in fact be the hallmark of most highly successful people). No, most people that are initially motivated by an idea never take the sufficient first steps to get off the line and see it through. This book follows a simple model to buck this trend[20] but we appreciate that any change in one's routine remains a big ask. Here are two simple ideas which might help build that extra layer of determination and allow you to embed the exercises quicker than you might think.

19: Peter M Gollwitzer, 'Implementation intentions – Strong Side Effects of Simple Plans', American Psychologist, July 1999
20: 1. Know the problem 2. How does this apply to me? 3. Simple everyday action

Make a Pledge

Making a pledge sounds much more daunting than it really needs to. No one is expecting you to raise one hand with the other on a Bible or take the Hippocratic Oath. Pledging in this context is about making your plans known to as many other people as possible. Your close family presumably know you are a snorer, and are likely snorers and future snorers themselves, so this is the best starting point. Given the types of domestic strain snoring causes this group are also likely to be a source of real support.

The basic theory says that the more people who know you are committed to making a change, the more likely you are to feel accountable and complete the journey. This is a very simple, almost obvious step to take but a study into marathon runners shows us that it is also incredibly effective. The study contained two focus groups of first-time marathon runners. Group one were left to their own devices and told only a small group of friends and family about their desire to complete the challenge. Group two were asked to pledge their intentions to as many people as possible. The results were stacked in favour of group two with nearly 85% of the participants completing a marathon within nine months of the pledge. Conversely 15% of group one had completed their set challenge, with the remainder presumably still "preparing".

Conditions are never perfect. The ducks will rarely align so stick your neck out and make a simple change that will have huge positive effects on your life and those around you.

Intentions

All best-made plans must reach the moment of action at some stage. Typically, this is the biggest hurdle in effective goal pursuit, however one that can be easily overcome if we understand the strong effects of simple plans.

We can all think of endless reasons not to do something – and the exercises above are no different. If you find it easy to put things off, or wait for non- rainy days then it is essential that you apply some basic intention theory to ensure that the activity gets completed. Try and focus on the routine one day at a time. Success will always be defined by the culmination of your daily activity and will prevent you from the influence of that niggling doubt or fear of the bigger picture.

Hopefully the option of being a non-snorer via such simple means is motivation enough but combined with a "take it each day as it comes" mentality you are on to a winning formula.

Finally, making good on your intentions and getting the activity done is evidence of becoming an expert in the field of how to stop snoring, expertise that others can benefit from. Evidence shows that people learn most through a combination of group discussion and teaching[21], so get out there and talk about your success and the massive changes that getting restful sleep has made to your personal and professional relationships, goals and aspirations.

.

21: *http://www.makeuseof.com/tag/10000-hour-rule-wrong-really-master-skill/*

Conclusion

The context for writing this book has always been a belief that people have more control over the factors that impact their lives than they give themselves credit for. Moreover, a lack of personal responsibility when it comes to health is leading to a nanny culture which is quite frankly unsustainable.

A huge burden is placed on society because of ailments, conditions and diseases that come about from voluntary habits. Beyond the campaigns against drug, tobacco and alcohol use we have argued that snoring in general should be added to this list.

Snoring and the lack of sufficient sleep it causes has been shown to affect the enjoyment of nearly every aspect of the personal and professional lives of its sufferers – not to mention the lives of those close to them.

Simple, effective and cost-neutral measures that we are each personally reasonable for must be the first response to breaking any voluntary habit. In the case of snoring the exercise routine we have designed will initially reduce the volume and frequency of snoring, leading to increasingly infrequent episodes and ultimately stopping the snoring altogether.

People make the change not prescriptions, pills or policy and you now have the keys to be the change you want to see in your own life.

END

About the Authors

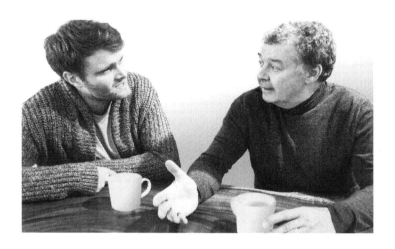

Mike Dilkes has been a consultant Ear, Nose and Throat surgeon in London's Harley Street for the last 20 years. Always at the for front of new developments in his field, he has innovated many new techniques over the years. He was the first in the UK to use lasers for hair removal and skin resurfacing, now everyday techniques. Mike is also the inventor of the Dilkes twin channel laser device. The treatment of snoring has always been of interest to him, and for many years has been researching new methods and ways of stopping snoring. This book is a culmination of long periods of analysis and thought as to the role of the throat muscles in snoring, and how modifying these structures can influence the severity of this condition.

Alexander Adams began his professional career as a clinical expert with GlaxoSmithKline. He has a talent for translating complex terminology into engaging formats which anyone can understand and benefit from – not just the healthcare professionals. As a specialist in a lifestyle and sustainable wellness, Alexander has a passion for cutting through the pseudo-science and is an ambassador for those simple, transformative health and fitness measures which make the biggest impact.